Robert G. Edwards:
A Personal Viewpoint

Joseph D. Schulman, M.D. © 2010

Dedicated to Robert G. Edwards, Ph.D., F.R.S.

Nobel Laureate in Physiology or Medicine 2010

The following is neither a comprehensive history of the development of in vitro fertilization (IVF), nor a full analysis of the careers of Nobel Laureate, Robert G. Edwards, Ph.D., F.R.S. or this writer. Rather, it is a highly personal rendition of events which the author participated in or witnessed relevant to the development of modern methods of assisted reproduction. It provides a true picture of the efforts and complexity behind a particular area of medical progress. The story also highlights challenges to innovation in the reproductive sciences and to moving these advances from the laboratory into widespread medical use.

Robert G. Edwards was finally, on October 4, 2010, awarded the Nobel Prize in Physiology and Medicine. The announcement from the Nobel Assembly at Sweden's Karolinska Institute is long overdue. Tragically, the recipient is in too poor condition to appreciate the award he so thoroughly deserves, as he is now 85 years old and for the past few years has been incapacitated by a progressive dementia.

It is my privilege to have Bob Edwards as a mentor and a friend for over 37 years. I also am one of the very few, and possibly the only person, still able to describe based on first-hand involvement certain aspects of the history of the very early development of human in-vitro fertilization pioneered by Bob, Patrick Steptoe, and

Jean Purdy. Much of what follows is absent from any published accounts on this subject.

I first learned about the British research on human embryos through an article not in the professional scientific literature but, somewhat remarkably, in a popular magazine. The writer reported the amazing news that a Ph.D. geneticist affiliated with Cambridge University, Dr. Robert G. Edwards, had actually formed human embryos from eggs and sperm in the laboratory. My recollection is that the report appeared in Harper's or the Atlantic Monthly. I saw it in 1968-69 while I was a pediatrician and post-doctoral biochemical genetics fellow at the National Institutes of Health in the section headed by J. Edwin ("Jay") Seegmiller, who later became a professor at U. Cal. – San Diego and a member of the National Academy of Sciences. My recent online search of the Harper's archives failed to locate the original article, and items from the Atlantic archives during the time period of relevance cannot be retrieved because of copyright restrictions.

I wasn't sure what to make of the lay report on Edward's work, but after reading what I could about it in the scientific literature discussed the subject with Jay and asked him what he thought about my trying to do embryo research with Edwards. Jay was aware that I had already decided that after finishing the NIH fellowship in 1970 I would enter a second medical specialty, obstetrics and gynecology, and continue my research on genetics – possibly on the NIH faculty – after this added clinical experience. Embryo genetics and infertility were new scientific frontiers that interested me. Jay kindly offered to check out Edwards through his professional contacts, and some time later reported to me that he was considered a respectable scientist.

I began a correspondence with Dr. Edwards to explore the possibility of coming to Cambridge to join his research team. He said that if I wanted to do this I would have to provide my own support, as he had no money available for this purpose. I suppose he thought that this would provide sufficient discouragement, and that he would hear from me no further. But that was not to be.

Upon leaving the NIH, I went to Cornell University Medical Center in New York, accompanied by my wife and two baby girls, and began my ob-gyn residency. I also continued research activities in genetics in collaboration with faculty in the obstetrics and pediatrics departments. The obstetrics chairman, Fritz Fuchs, encouraged my research interests, and appreciated that I had been a productive scientist while at NIH where I had even been given the rare opportunity to run a laboratory independently after Seegmiller left to take a professorship in California. Fritz was a pioneer in the field of prenatal genetics. While still in Denmark he had performed the world's first testing of fetuses for gender via amniocentesis and Barr body analysis (microscopically examining amniotic fluid cells for the "inactive" X chromosome found only in cells from females), with the aim of preventing X-linked disease such as hemophilia and Duchenne muscular dystrophy. The chairman of pediatrics, Wallace McCrory, also welcomed my working with his department on genetic problems. Dr. Fuchs even helped provide a tiny laboratory space for my work on amino acid analysis in amniotic fluid. I also collaborated with John Queenan, later to become chairman of Ob-Gyn at Georgetown University, on amniotic fluid chemistry and fetal Rh disease, and began a long friendship with future obstetrical geneticist and U. Texas – Houston department chairman Joe Leigh Simpson.

Busy as I was with other things, I kept my eye on the possibility of locating funds to work with Edwards. Everyone I spoke to said it sounded exciting, but money for study abroad on human embryo research seemed non-existent, and family circumstances did not permit private funding of such an effort. Then I got lucky. At one of the clinics in New York Hospital I met Dr. Virginia Apgar. She was the inventor of the widely utilized "Apgar score" for assessing the wellbeing of babies immediately after birth, and had become active in the National Foundation – March of Dimes. She either then was or would soon become its President. The March of Dimes was, of course, founded to raise money for polio research, but the virtual elimination of polio after development of the vaccine by Jonas Salk and then an improved vaccine by Albert Sabin had forced a change in the direction of the Foundation's research. Its Board had decided to focus on research on genetic disorders – an important and farsighted decision. Dr. Apgar was excited to learn that I was active in genetics and took a liking to me. As we talked, I told her about my dream of getting to England to work with Edwards on embryonic genetics. By this time, I had already been offered a faculty position to return to the National Institutes of Health in 1974. My residency ended in mid-1973. So approximately one year in Cambridge could be managed in 1973-74. I told Virginia I thought it would then be possible to return to NIH and continue working on both human genetics and human embryology. She offered to see if she could persuade the March of Dimes to provide some support for my going abroad.

A few weeks later, Dr. Apgar had lined up a grant of $10,000 to support my working with Bob Edwards. I was most grateful for her help. But these were insufficient funds to finance a year in Cambridge for a family of four, during which my pediatrician wife would not be allowed to work in England as a physician due to licensing restrictions. Fortunately, I became aware that Harvard Medical School, where I had received my medical degree, offered something called a Gilbert Traveling

Fellowship, sponsored by a former HMS graduate who felt that future American scientists would benefit from contact with research activities in Europe. The fellowship was specifically for study abroad for one year, and paid a stipend of approximately $9,000. I applied for and received the Gilbert Fellowship conditional, as the March of Dimes award also was, upon my being formally accepted to do research with Edwards at Cambridge. The combination of the two sources of support seemed just enough to cover anticipated travel and living expenses.

I believe Bob Edwards was surprised to learn that I really had found the money to come to his laboratory, and that he felt morally obligated to say "Yes", which he did. Thus it was that with his consent and the awards from Harvard and March of Dimes my family and I sailed from New York to Southampton in late August, 1973, and then proceeded by train to Cambridge.

We had arranged to rent a house on Queen Edith's Way near the southern fringe of Cambridge. Fairly spacious by British standards, the house was two stories high with a back garden containing apple trees and littered with fallen apples which had never been collected. It was heated by a circulating hot water system which later failed in mid-winter, and which our lease as well as the freezing cold required us to repair at substantial cost. A single phone was placed inconveniently in the kitchen, far from the upstairs bedrooms; we discovered that the Postal Service provides the telephones in England and that the waiting time to get an extension or a second phone line installed was over one year. We acquired a used Rover sedan from a friendly but dishonest young couple who presented an MOT (Ministry of Transport) certificate stating that the car had passed inspection. After purchasing the vehicle we discovered that it was unexpectedly a gas hog, were shocked that a liter of gasoline cost about as much in Great Britain as a full gallon in the U.S., and were even more distressed to learn that one of the car's four cylinders was not working – which was obviously why the lemon had been sold - and that fixing it would consume over one thousand dollars of our extremely limited funds. We were, to borrow a phrase, typical Innocents Abroad.

But the excitement of being in England and looking forward to starting with Edwards in mid-September were more than sufficient compensation for these practical challenges. Our little girls were registered in the local schools, which for some reason required that "Wellingtons" (waterproof boots of a type perhaps worn during the Battle of Waterloo) had to be purchased for them by their parents as a requirement of attendance. Wellingtons proved useful not only in rain, but also on ice and snow, and the kids frequently wore them to school. The city of Cambridge is located in East Anglia, which as we later discovered is one of the coldest parts of England. Natives claim that the winter winds cross unimpeded over the North Sea straight from Russia. Winter also brings darkness. We learned the implications of living at the latitude of central Labrador as in mid-winter the sun feebly dissipated the darkness at close to 9 AM, skimmed low across the usually cloudy sky, and then descended below the horizon at about 3 PM to start another long, frigid night. Cambridge is, of course, lovely in the fall and spring when it is not raining – but it rains there a lot too. Living in England was to give us a particular appreciation of the climatic reasons why it was deemed desirable that the sun never set on the British Empire, and why the Brits were attracted in their colonial heyday to such hot, sunny locations as India and the deserts of the Middle East.

Cambridge University is a collection of mostly grey stone Gothic-style structures scattered throughout the city, with a particular concentration along the banks of the tiny River Cam. The Cam is delightful for "punting" (poling along in a small boat), and its green banks are the site of much undergraduate repose. Some of the most famous of the old buildings, like King's College chapel, are impressively lovely. The newer postwar colleges are not particularly attractive, and I had been assigned a dining affiliation (rarely used since the food was so bad) and temporary membership in one of the newest, Darwin College.

The Marshall Laboratory where I at last went to meet Bob Edwards was located on the top floor of the Physiological Laboratory building, one of a closely packed warren of dark brick buildings near Downing Street. Compared to the facilities at Harvard and the NIH the labs looked rather dingy, small, and minimally equipped. One lower floor of the building was largely occupied by a common room in which the inescapable rituals of "morning coffee" (mid-morning) and "afternoon tea" were daily shared by all. The Marshall Lab itself was mostly one fairly spacious experimentation room shared by several of the graduate students, to which my presence was then added. There were a few smaller lab spaces, and compact offices for the faculty. The head of the unit was C.R. ("Bunny") Austin, who served as department chairman and was a full professor at Cambridge. Bunny was from Australia, and had published an interesting book on the mammalian oocyte in addition to his peer-reviewed scientific work. He was a warm, friendly man and strongly in favor of the work Bob Edwards was doing with human embryos. I liked him immediately. He introduced me to Bob.

Bob Edwards, then a Reader (associate professor), occupied a tiny office overflowing with irregular stacks of papers. There was space in the room for no more than two chairs, with him in one of them. He was casually dressed and had a wonderful smile. My first impression was of a dynamic, very high level of energy. He was quick and enthusiastic in speech and gesture. It soon became apparent that his grasp of the science of both animal and human reproduction was encyclopedic, and indeed I have never met anyone who knew as much about these subjects as Bob. I later got to attend some of his brilliant lectures on reproduction to students at Cambridge.

We talked little about human IVF at our initial meeting. Bob explained that the human IVF work took place only in the winter and spring, after his teaching responsibilities were finished in the fall semester, and he seemed to prefer to discuss IVF later on. I agreed to work on a laboratory project involving animals in the interim. Bob had gotten his Ph.D. in animal genetics, was aware of my own genetic experience, and he tried to direct me toward a study of the cytogenetics of meiosis (gamete formation) in the mouse. He had worked in this area some years ago, and felt that extensions of his experiments could add useful knowledge. This type of study would have been rather far removed from my personal interests and my past research in genetics related to biochemistry and genetic diseases, and after thinking it over I really did not want to do it. We agreed that I could instead develop my own research plan, provided costs were only modest for what I proposed, and I began a project involving the examination of biochemical changes during implantation of the early embryo in the wall of the uterus with particular regard to an enzyme, gamma-glutamyl transpeptidase, thought to be related to amino acid transport. I also supplemented this research with quite different studies which I carried out one to two days per week in London at the Children's Hospital on Great Ormond Street with my friend, A. Desmond ("Des") Patrick, who like me had been actively engaged in research on cystinosis, a genetic disease primarily of children. I became quite familiar with the long train ride between Cambridge and London's St. Pancras terminal near the Children's Hospital which started in wintertime while the moon was still in the sky and the sun nowhere to be seen. Some of my time in London was also spent in the reading room of the British Museum, learning about antique maps the collection of which in these days, when they were extraordinarily inexpensive, could be pursued better in London than anywhere else.

At the Marshall, I was turned over to the graduate students (Bob's, Bunny's, and those of another faculty member, Dennis New) to guide me on the practical aspects of how the lab functioned, and of course to learn the scuttlebutt of what was really going on. The Ph.D. candidates in the lab included some very talented young scientists. Among them were Azim Surani, later to become famous for his pioneering work on genetic imprinting, Martin Johnson, David Cockroft, Pat Coppola, and Richard Gardner. Gardner, a future professor at Oxford, amazed me by his uncanny ability to cannulate tiny structures, such as the oviducts of living mice, without traumatic bleeding under a dissecting microscope – he would have made a brilliant surgeon. Cockroft seemed quiet and mostly kept to himself. Pat helped me with several experiments. Johnson, who is a professor today at Cambridge, told me that Edwards' work on human IVF had "no scientific merit", but he has, of course, greatly changed this youthful view. Barry Bavister, who helped developed one of the culture media then used in the human IVF work and had shared with Bob the thrill of achieving in Cambridge in 1969 the first fertilizations of human eggs in vitro, had finished his graduate work and I never got to meet him at the Marshall. Roger Gosden was a tall, shy graduate student who was always pleasant to me, and he later did important innovative work on freezing and reimplanting of ovarian tissue in animals. Like Bavister, Roger later migrated to the United States.

It seemed that of this exceptionally talented group of grad students none of them had ever been allowed to visit the little hospital at Oldham (Dr. Kershaw's Cottage Hospital was its original name) outside of Manchester where the human IVF work including embryo replacements into patients was now being carried out. I am sure most of them doubted I would ever get there either.

My research on implantation-related enzyme histochemistry proceeded in Cambridge, and I greatly enjoyed my days in London with biochemist

Des Patrick, a most loveable and brilliant man. Also, my family and I took American-style revenge against a British government that had betrayed Israel during the recent Yom Kippur War in the Middle East. We had been deeply upset about the war, resented the biased statements about it by British spokesmen at Whitehall including Foreign Secretary Alex Douglas-Home, and were horrified when England violated its prior agreement to supply critical shells for Israel's Chieftain tanks. During 1973-74, Britain was beset by crises including a shortage of imported oil (there was no North Sea oil in those days), a national coal miner strike, and a national railroad worker strike. We gleefully violated the government's voluntary guidelines on energy conservation; in our otherwise darkened Cambridge neighborhood all the lights in our home shone brightly, and on weekends we enjoyed taking long drives in the countryside and down to London on highways made nearly empty by responsible Brits who, in marked contrast to ourselves, were staying off the roads as requested by Prime Minister Edward Heath. My wife and I were, on a single occasion, invited to Bob Edward's home, where we met his gracious wife, Ruth Fowler - herself a Ph.D. and early collaborator on some of Bob's research with ovulation induction in animals - and several of their five daughters, as well as the well-known reproductive scientist, Alan Parkes. I learned to adapt to the Marshall Lab's scientists' usual schedule, which involved rarely coming to work before about 10 AM, then breaking for morning coffee, taking little or no lunch, breaking for afternoon tea, and working on as long as necessary and commonly until the wee hours of the morning. I was having an interesting time in a stimulating environment. But as the winter seriously set in, Bob had still not proposed when we were going to Oldham, nor had we had much discussion about his human IVF research.

Sometime near the end of 1973, I brought up the subject of IVF again and asked Bob when we were going to start at Oldham. I had not yet met Patrick Steptoe, who was up in Manchester, and had only briefly been introduced to Jean Purdy, the nurse who also served as the IVF technician at Oldham and who, although she lived in Cambridge, did only limited work at the Marshall Lab. I was eager to get started. But Bob had other ideas. He proposed that I just stay in Cambridge and continue my research on animals during the winter and spring, and not go to Oldham. I became angry. Restraining myself as best I could I expressed feelingly to Bob that working on IVF was the very reason that I had come to England. I no longer recall exactly what I said, but it included stating that I was a fairly senior scientist, not a graduate student; I had made a major financial sacrifice to come to Cambridge on a fellowship stipend instead of drawing a salary at NIH which was probably larger than Bob himself was receiving at this University; I was a respected American scientist who fully shared his vision that IVF was going to be of great importance; and he had made commitments to me before I had come to England which I felt he had an obligation to fulfill. To my surprise, he did not blow up and seemed taken aback by my vigorous comments. He then said something like, "I will talk to Patrick and get back to you."

And he did. A few days later, he told me that I was welcome to come to Oldham with him and Jean, and to meet Patrick. The first trip was only a few days away. I warmly thanked Bob, and shared the good news with my wife. At last, I was about to enter the inner sanctum.

Only over time did I come to understand the various reasons for the secrecy that surrounded the human IVF effort, a seclusion contrasting with the openness typically presumed to occur in serious university-based scientific activities. I never directly discussed the reasons for this with Bob. One obvious factor was that Bob and Patrick wanted to be the first to produce a baby through IVF. They knew that after the publication of Bob's 1969 paper demonstrating fertilization of human eggs outside the body other teams were competing with them, and these teams (primarily in Australia) had some very smart folks on board, people whom I later got to know personally like Alex Lopata, Alan Trounson, Ian Johnston, and Carl Wood. Bob was realistic enough to know too that in the race to publish new science, participants were not always completely scrupulous about utilizing and publishing other people's ideas - and if such ideas or their scientific details are not discussed or published they are much harder to co-opt. At the time I had not experienced such co-opting, but subsequently I learned in a highly personal way that it really does happen. Some years later when I was on the faculty at NIH I conceived, in association with Mort Lipsett and others, the use of a steroid called dexamethasone for prevention of abnormal genital masculinization in female fetuses with congenital adrenal hyperplasia (CAH); our work was being written up for publication when I mentioned it to an endocrinologist in France, who shared our information with a French academician working on this genetic disease. While anonymous reviewers delayed publication of our study, this latter person published ahead of us, thus ensuring her own scientific credit for our discovery. And even then I did not learn. While running our own Institute and already past the age of 50, by which time I should have known better, I told a visiting professor from England that we had observed a high frequency of ovarian insufficiency in carriers of another genetic disease, Fragile X syndrome; this lady hastily published a series of such cases ahead of us, gave us no credit in that publication, and is today generally considered to be the discoverer of premature ovarian failure in Fragile X females.

But there were additional reasons for Bob's secrecy. I was aware that his efforts actually to produce an IVF baby were considered controversial and even dangerous by some people, but I had only a limited appreciation at that time of just how awful the controversy was. Bob had been repeatedly attacked by the sensationalist British press. He had been vilified by religious leaders of the Catholic Church and - even more importantly in England - some but not all leaders of the Anglican Church. Colleagues at Cambridge, including the Nobel Laureate Max Perutz, had spoken angrily to Bob about the dangers of what he was trying to do. He was accused of running the risk of making malformed monster babies. His research funding from the Medical Research Council (MRC), the British equivalent of the NIH, was threatened. False accusations about Bob's work were so extreme that he later had to issue successful libel actions to silence them. Some of his own graduate students were opposed to what he was attempting, and were intimidated from participation by negative opinions from more senior scientists. The atmosphere is captured in the following fascinating admission, which can now be seen online, by Professor Martin Johnson in association with a conference on IVF in 2009:

"If I'm honest, while we were doing our PhDs, and even into our postdoctoral time in the lab, both Richard [Gardner] and I were very unsure about whether what Bob was doing was appropriate, and we didn't want to get too involved in it. The reasons for that were partly because it was quite unsettling as graduate students and early postdocs to see the sheer level of hostility to the work - when Nobel Laureates and the Fellows of the Royal Society and the emerging bigwigs of the subject like Bob Winston and Roger Short were lambasting into Bob and saying, you shouldn't do it... you had to say, well, what's going on here? Can one man be right against this weight of authoritative opinion? ....Numerous people were saying, why is a man like Bob wasting his time on a trivial problem like infertility, which isn't really important to anyone? I remember this coming again and again and again from other scientists, people I respected could be totally dismissive and scathing about Bob, saying he's lovely man, but completely misguided …. he really shouldn't be doing this work because it's immoral as well as a waste of his talent. That was the general theme. We were in this sort of little ghetto at the top of Physiology, which was ringed with prejudice and hostility and antagonism...............How short sighted we were! And what a remarkable visionary Bob was."

Or, as Bob's department head, "Bunny" Austin expressed it with significantly greater understatement after Bob won the Lasker Award in 1991:

"Bob became involved with vigorous and often heated debate on moral and ethical issues as well as on the medical and biological ones.......The intense public interest was steadfastly maintained....."

Thus, in 1973 Bob Edwards was feeling the pressures of rejection of his vision by many fellow scientists. But now had arrived, from across the Atlantic, a true believer, a supporter both morally and scientifically, a recognized medical investigator and prospective NIH faculty member who shared Bob's dream and did not doubt its rightness. Perhaps more than any other factors, these may explain why Bob allowed me - and, to my knowledge, nobody else before the birth of Louise Brown, the world's first IVF baby - to participate in the efforts by him, Patrick, and Jean in Oldham. Once Bob and Patrick had made that decision, numerous discussions on IVF began between Bob and me; the barriers were removed, and we exchanged ideas with complete frankness. Needless to say, I learned far more from these discussions than Bob did, but he seemed to like to bounce his ideas off me and enjoyed these exchanges. He was particularly focused, as was the whole team, on one major question: Why were the seemingly normal embryos which they had been able to produce from more than a few of Patrick's patients consistently failing to implant and produce an ongoing pregnancy after replacement in the uterus?

The morning came to pick up Jean Purdy in our rented Ford and head up toward Manchester. Jean was about thirty years of age, sandy haired, fairly attractive, invariably friendly, enthusiastic and tremendously devoted to Bob and the IVF project. Jean and I got along well, and I was shocked to learn of her untimely death from cancer in the 1980s. She was the only person other than Bob, and later myself, who actually knew all the details of the team's IVF laboratory methodology and participated in making the culture media and handling the eggs and embryos; she also doubled as the IVF team's only nurse. We always used Ford cars for these long drives, and Bob told me it was because the Ford Foundation had provided part of the funding for the team's IVF research. I had the dubious distinction of sitting in the front left seat (the British "death seat") while Bob sped us up the A1 motorway toward the North. To reach the Manchester area (the tiny hospital where the IVF work was done was actually in Royton, a suburb of Oldham, which was in turn a suburb of Manchester) one had to cross to the west of England over the Pennine mountains on either the M62 motorway or over secondary roads. Royton was close to the M62 and we often drove by this route but it was longer than if one cut across the mountains on the smaller roads. Bob preferred the more direct route over the mountains unless the weather was bad. He was a fast and skillful driver, but I felt he trusted that skill a little too much on several occasions. I recall one truly hair-raising trip over the Pennines in a snowstorm with Bob barely slowly down on the icy curves while Jean cowered in the back and I imagined my life ending then and there.

We had dinner with Patrick Steptoe and his beautiful wife, Sheena, at an upscale restaurant in Manchester. Sheena had been an actress on the London stage, and she and Patrick met when he was supporting himself during medical school playing live piano to accompany theatrical performances. I liked Sheena very much, and it was among the many tragedies affecting the IVF team that she developed a debilitating stroke shortly after the birth of Louise Brown in 1978. Patrick himself died of prostate cancer in 1988. I never got to see Patrick's home, but I often was able to admire the magnificent 12 cylinder crimson Jaguar sedan in which he was known to zoom down to London at over 100 miles per hour. Patrick was a self-confident, sophisticated man with distinguished grey hair and intelligent eyes, and wearing first-rate London custom tailoring. He looked like the highly successful surgeon he was (professionally he was called, in the British manner, "Mr. Steptoe", not "Doctor Steptoe"). An excellent listener, he spoke less than Bob but what he said always made good sense. He was the only person I knew who could actually tell Bob Edwards to shut up. In fact, during our dinner together I recall Patrick saying to Bob, "You told me Joe was an intelligent guy. I'd like to hear what *he* thinks."

Patrick was far more than just a successful practitioner. He was a medical pioneer hardened by controversy and well-known long before he got involved in IVF-related investigations. Trained as a surgeon, he was the first in England to appreciate the importance of a new technique for visualizing the contents of a sick patient's abdomen without the need for a large surgical incision. This method, called diagnostic laparoscopy, had been developed by Raoul Palmer in Paris. Steptoe understood the importance of laparoscopy, went to Paris, learned the technique from Palmer, and brought it back to England. Its introduction into British medicine was difficult. It threatened some established ways of doing surgery, and was resisted by conservative surgeons. Before fiberoptic instrumentation was developed, viewing intra-abdominal contents through a laparoscope required the introduction of a small light bulb into the abdomen, and there was a risk of burns from the bulb. Laparoscopy also, even today, involves a low risk of perforation of an intra-abdominal organ before or during introduction of the scope. And, of course, laparoscopy was a "foreign" technique developed by a Frenchman. Although Patrick's efforts to do laparoscopy for gynecological disorders in England met considerable initial resistance, he doggedly persisted, lecturing and demonstrating his methods in many hospitals. Eventually laparoscopy won acceptance because it is far easier and safer for patients than major surgery. Steptoe's small book on laparoscopy became a minor medical classic, and helped him earn the sobriquet "The Father of British Laparoscopy".

Bob Edwards had been looking for a non-surgical method of obtaining human eggs for IVF studies. He attended one of Patrick's lectures and thought that laparoscopy could be the best available way to safely recover eggs. He discussed this with Patrick who, always quick to understand and appreciate good ideas, enthusiastically became Bob's research partner and eventually his close friend. Patrick's interest in innovations in medicine continued until his death at age 75. In fact, although he was a pioneer in laparoscopy and IVF cycles both in England and the United States were initially performed with the aid of laparoscopy, one of Patrick's last publications shortly before his death was on ultrasound-guided egg retrieval for IVF, a method pioneered by Pierre Dellenbach in Strasbourg and by myself in the U.S. and which came to entirely replace the obtaining of eggs via laparoscopy.

Upon arrival at the tiny hospital near Oldham, which had, as I recall about twenty beds, two of which were reserved for IVF patients, I was directed to sleep in a miniscule room with a cot near the single operating room and the adjacent IVF lab. The nearest bathroom was far away at the end of a long, dimly lit hallway. The only two decent rooms for overnight habitation were, of course, already occupied by Bob and Jean and were located on the floor above. Patrick never stayed overnight at the hospital. But the rest of us usually spent 3-4 days there on each of the approximately 15 trips we made to Royton from Cambridge in the winter and spring of 1974.

The simplicity of the IVF facilities at the hospital was extreme. The laboratory was about 7 feet deep and 12 feet wide. It had a single door and no window. It contained a hood with filtered air flow, within which was a low power binocular Wild microscope, and a higher powered inverted phase-contrast microscope for close examination of fertilization and cleavage in living embryos. A round, portable glass chamber about 18 inches across, with a valve for controlling the inflow of a 5% carbon dioxide - 95% air mixture, also sat in the hood ready for connection when needed to a tank of the compressed gas. To the right and outside the hood was a steel incubator maintained at a temperature of 37 degrees Centigrade. Within this was to be placed the gassed, glass chamber within which the eggs were incubated with sperm, and subsequently the early embryos further incubated until they had divided into several cells and were ready for replacement in the uterus. To the left of the hood and above it were shelves containing the chemical ingredients for making the culture media, and a laboratory balance for careful weighing of these chemicals. The total cost of the equipment in that tiny lab was probably less than $10,000 dollars. The "theatre" in the hospital looked like a typical operating room with overhead surgical lights and a surgical table beneath it. Steptoe's laparoscope, a relatively new fiberoptic instrument with its external light source, stood nearby. And that was it! The total space occupied could not have been more than 600 square feet (including my sleeping room). Here was important science being done with simple equipment, minimal budget, a team of three persons with great energy and determination to which my own efforts were now being added, directed by one giant brain pursuing a goal that would make possible the birth of millions of babies. To me, the whole thing was deeply inspiring. I also believed that this very year we would achieve the first successful IVF pregnancy.

I assisted Bob and Jean in the making and gaseous equilibrating of fresh culture media (two slightly different ones were utilized, one for fertilizing the eggs, and the other for embryos). Soon our first laparoscopy was underway. Patrick always did these himself, with me assisting. He was surprised that I already knew how to do laparoscopy, but in fact Cornell had its own pioneer in diagnostic laparoscopy, Dr. William Sweeney, and I had learned laparoscopic technique from Bill during my residency in New York City. Nevertheless, only Patrick ever operated on Patrick's patients. He did permit me to look through the laparoscope from time to time, to observe the ovarian bulges (the fluid-filled follicles containing eggs) which he aspirated under direct vision using a gentle suction device. This fluid was immediately brought to the lab by Jean, and Bob would then decant the liquid into Petri dishes and examine it for eggs under the Wild scope. Viable eggs were then transferred into smaller Petri dishes containing gas-equilibrated sterile medium, and a washed, diluted sample of the husband's semen was added. The dishes were then covered, placed into the portable glass covered vessel which was re-gassed and then place overnight in the incubator.

The next day, the eggs were examined by Bob (and later by me or Bob) for evidence of fertilization, the presence of small round pronuclei within the eggs. In most of the patients, at least one of the eggs did fertilize. I do not recall the proportion of fertilized eggs which, on average, then underwent normal cleavage into early-stage embryos, but I believe that in about half of the patients one or more embryos reached the stage at which they could be replaced into the uterus. This was either done via a laparoscopically-guided needle through the abdomen or using a fine catheter threaded through the natural opening of the cervix.

I can, of course, vividly remember my excitement at being one of the first people in the world to observe living human eggs and embryos! It seemed an enormous privilege and responsibility to be doing this. I never grew tired of the sight, and neither apparently did Bob. When he saw a healthy looking embryo he would rave enthusiastically, "A beauty! Beautiful! Joe, come look at this." I learned quickly that a "beautiful" embryo was round with a symmetrical pattern of cleavage, filling the space within the "shell" (zona pellucida) surrounding the embryo; these were the embryos which were thought to be the most normal and able to establish pregnancies.

But although we tried week after week through most of the winter and spring, sometimes with one, two, or three infertile patients per week, no pregnancy resulted. About 30 embryo transfer procedures were carried out. We extensively debated the possible causes of failure, of which the informed scientific imagination could provide many. Bob and I spent hours talking about this alone, sometimes with Jean or with Patrick. Nobody could be sure that the culture conditions were not inhibiting the health of the embryos. Most of the patients had received a fertility drug called clomiphene citrate ("Clomid") to stimulate the production of more than one egg per treatment cycle, with final egg ripening hours before laparoscopy catalyzed by an injection of a hormone called HCG. Bob felt that clomiphene was safe to use in IVF, since this drug had helped patients who did not have blocked Fallopian tubes to achieve pregnancies without IVF. He also believed that aspiration of the follicles might inhibit formation of the corpus luteum, a progesterone-producing body that appears in the ovary post-ovulation and which is needed to sustain pregnancy; for this reason all our patients received additional progestational supplementation via injection of a synthetic progesterone analogue, Primulot. Nobody could be sure if these drugs were helping, or perhaps unnecessary or even having adverse consequences. We also were uncertain about the best way to insert embryos back into the uterus, and speculated that even minimal trauma to the endometrial lining of the uterus might be blocking implantation.

As the experimental efforts continued, and still none of the embryos produced pregnancies, we felt growing disappointment and a premonition of failure. The effect on Bob was particularly severe. The strain he was under was enormous. His scientific credibility and integrity were being questioned by many scientists and members of the public. Although it was never disclosed it to me at time, Bunny Austin has subsequently revealed that the project's sources of support were about to end. Indeed, the IVF efforts in the next three years before the first pregnancy happened received financing from Steptoe's private practice. As patient after patient failed to conceive, Bob, never the most patient of men, became increasingly irritable. On our last departure together from Oldham tension caused him to lose his temper over a trivial comment I had made, and the rest of the drive back to Cambridge was accomplished in a mutually awkward silence, which an embarrassed Jean also hesitated to break.

A few weeks later, I concluded my animal experiments in Cambridge, paid a last visit to Des Patrick in London, and prepared to return to the

United States and start my work at NIH. I left on friendly terms with Bob, Bunny, and the rest of the crowd at the Marshall. I believe Jean was particularly sorry to see me go. She also was upset at the immense strain Bob was under. Better than anyone except perhaps Bob's wife, Ruth, she seemed to empathize with his depth of disappointment. I and my family, and the precious laboratory notebook in which I had recorded all the details of the IVF clinical and laboratory methods, flew back to Washington. I still have that notebook, which is intended to be donated to a museum of science.

Thus we come to the end of my year of doing IVF research in England. But that is hardly the end of our story. The future was filled with many surprises.

Their personal history of the IVF effort, published by Bob and Patrick for the general public after the birth of Louise Brown, provides only the briefest history of the dark period of repetitive failure from 1972 when the first embryo replacements were done through 1975; indeed, it is hardly mentioned at all, nor by the way is my presence at Royton or Cambridge. This period is truly the "black hole" of the history of IVF, a time about which little information has emerged. In fact, despite his incredible toughness and tenacity, Bob briefly became sufficiently discouraged that he attempted to pursue a career as a Labor Party politician, but he was fortunately defeated and thereafter continued his research to the great benefit of mankind. With financing from Patrick's practice and perhaps from other undisclosed sources, the work in Oldham went on. Attempts were made to achieve pregnancies using frozen embryos, even donor embryos, because it was thought that the process of egg removal might interfere with natural processes necessary for pregnancy attainment. Finally, totally natural cycles without any medications were attempted, harvesting only a single egg and timing the laparoscopy by monitoring the natural rise of the hormone LH before ovulation. A tubal pregnancy resulted, which somewhat later was followed by the successful initiation in 1977 of the pregnancy that resulted in the 1978 birth of Louise Brown.

Today, very few IVF treatments use natural menstrual cycles, which are less efficient in establishing pregnancies than correctly performed drug-stimulated cycles. Why did the natural cycles finally work in Oldham? Bob told me and others that he believes it was because the drug used for luteal phase support, Primulot, actually destroyed the patient's own capacity to sustain a corpus luteum, causing a kind of very early abortion of the pregnancy. This may be the whole explanation, or there may be other factors including improvements in the purity of IVF reagents which also made Louise Brown possible. I recall debating with Bob about using natural progesterone in oil instead of

Primulot; he felt they would have equivalent effects but that repeated injections of progesterone in oil would be too uncomfortable for patients. Those familiar with IVF methods will know that Bob's concern about progesterone in oil was exaggerated, as this agent has subsequently been used in thousands of IVF cycles without major difficulty.

The immense success marked by the birth of Louise Brown led Bob to expect that the British government-funded health care system would provide resources for the clinical delivery of IVF services to infertile couples. But his then Laborite faith in government-sponsored health care was shockingly disappointed. The government hospital system, concerned about costs, refused to provide any resources or funds for IVF treatments. In retrospect, and using modern parlance, this was an early example of the rationing of care and innovation which has become a prominent part of many socialized health care systems including those of Canada and Great Britain. All else failing, Bob was driven into the "private sector". He and Patrick located two principal investors, and together they purchased Bourn Hall, a country estate near Cambridge which was converted to a combined short-stay hospital and outpatient clinic for the delivery of IVF services to self-paying patients. Very quickly thereafter Bourn Hall was treating a large number of infertile couples from all over the world. Bob, Patrick, and their team pioneered numerous clinical improvements in IVF technology and achieved thousands of IVF pregnancies. As Bob told me later, after Patrick died in 1988 it became less enjoyable for him to be doing IVF. Bourn Hall was then sold that same year to Serono, a manufacturer of fertility drugs, for an undisclosed sum which, as Bob recounted it, was the *lowest* offer the owners had received for its acquisition.

Thus Bob achieved a degree of financial comfort almost despite himself, and it became possible for him and Ruth to retire to a farm outside Cambridge. He officially retired his professorship at Cambridge University in 1989, but his incredible energy made a mockery of the word "retirement". Always a voracious reader of the scientific literature and a fine writer of it as well, he edited the journal, "Human Reproduction", published by the European Society of Human Reproduction and Embryology (ESHRE), and turned it into the world's finest journal in the field of infertility. Later, Bob resigned that editorship and started his own, competing entirely electronic journal called RBM Online. Not surprisingly it became quite successful, sometimes publishing better science more quickly than ESHRE's journal. This doubtless lost some friends for Bob within the European reproductive medicine hierarchy.

While the editor of both Human Reproduction and RBM Online, and as the great reproductive pioneer he was, Bob spoke out strongly in favor of the important development by

Dr. Larry Johnson, I, and others at the Genetics & IVF Institute of the method of preconceptual gender selection known as MicroSort. Appropriately utilized, MicroSort enhances reproductive options and prevents genetic diseases while reducing gender-related abortions. But, as it had concerning IVF itself, the British health care bureaucracy continued to ignore Bob's advice, also was unresponsive to favorable recommendations from a special Parliamentary committee, and MicroSort technology is not currently available for patients in England.

Bob thus managed to offend some of his fellow academicians by prospering as a "capitalist", and antagonized the bureaucrats in his country's health care system over both IVF and MicroSort. These actions contributed substantially to the long delay in Bob's receipt of the Nobel Prize.

There continued to be a common thread in the history of Bob's later career and my own, and a digression is required. I had returned to NIH in 1974 planning to continue my research on genetic diseases and begin America's first IVF program for infertility treatment and research in the newly established clinical wing of the National Institute of Child Health and Human Development in Bethesda. In fact, an operating room suitable for laparoscopic egg retrievals had actually been built at NIH for this purpose. But then, like the British government, the American government put its foot in its mouth over

IVF, though in a different way. In August, 1974, just a few months after I started working as an NIH faculty member, and without any preliminary discussion with me or other informed reproductive scientists, the Secretary of Health and Human Services, who at that time was the Republican appointee Casper Weinberger, placed a moratorium on federal funding for IVF research. This shocking bureaucratic action could only have resulted as an extension of the "controversy" surrounding the efforts being made at Oldham, and an awareness that I was planning to begin similar work at the NIH. The moratorium was said not to be a permanent ban; rather, it was presented as a temporary measure which would be followed by public hearings to see if the moratorium should be lifted. This was extremely disappointing, but as I enjoyed great satisfaction at NIH from my other research activities in genetics I initially chose to remain at my faculty position there. In 1974 it of course seemed possible that IVF might never be successful clinically. And, I reasoned, if it did succeed in England or Australia the NIH would then surely be able to proceed with subsequent IVF research which would obviously be needed. For the next four years, however, no hearings took place and the ban remained.

    Like Bob, I had underestimated the relentless folly of our respective government officials. When Louise Brown was born, HHS finally was forced to create an advisory panel to evaluate the suitability of U.S. government funding of IVF research. The Chairman of that panel was handpicked by then HHS Secretary, the Democrat appointee Joseph Califano. The Chairman, a lawyer friend of Califano's, was anticipated to be deeply conservative on reproductive issues. The panel was selectively populated with Catholics, conservative Democrats, religious leaders, and handpicked friends such as the wife of the legendary Washington attorney, Edward Bennett Williams. It was not difficult to believe that the intention of the Secretary was that the committee report negatively about IVF research.

    The panel held most of its hearings on the NIH campus, and I was among the experts who appeared before it. Bob Edwards was invited to speak before the group, and he declined. He also advised me, privately and rather pointedly, that I must not attempt to speak for him or represent his views to the panel. I told the committee of my views that IVF was a wonderful breakthrough for infertile couples, it was strongly pro-family and "pro-life", and that federally funded research programs were important and would help to improve IVF further. I was impressed with the intelligence and questions of the panel members, and none of them revealed any hostility toward what I had been saying. Some months later, to Califano's surprise as he reported years later in his autobiography, the panel report strongly supported federal funding of IVF research. My recollection is that at least 10 members of the panel, including the Chairman, were in favor, and only two expressed limited reservations. And interestingly, a close relative of one of the panel members actually became an IVF patient of mine a few years later.

Califano's autobiography somehow fails to mention what happened after the panel's favorable report reached him. The committee was technically advisory to the Secretary. This meant that he could accept or reject its recommendations, modify them, or defer action on them. Califano chose to do absolutely nothing - he pigeonholed the report, and the moratorium continued. And it has subsequently remained in place through multiple changes of the Presidency, numerous Secretaries of HHS, and many alterations in the balances of power in Congress. It is amazing but true that although the NIH has repeatedly solicited HHS for approval to begin to fund IVF research, in fact has done so with most if not all changes in the Administration, such approval has never been granted. The moratorium on federal funding of IVF-related science continues to this day, over 35 years after Weinberger, now long deceased, initiated it, and even after several million IVF babies have been born around the world!

The birth of Louise Brown and the persistent failure of the NIH to be authorized to fund IVF research were game changers for me. I wanted to be part of the medical leadership which would bring

IVF into the world and make significant improvements in it. With some regrets and trepidation, I left the NIH and started one of America's first IVF programs at a university in Washington, DC where I was simultaneously a professor of obstetrics and gynecology. But there I quickly grew unhappy over the circumstances in which I had to work. Like Bob Edwards, I decided to go out into the cold, into the academically-despised "private sector." Thus the Genetics & IVF Institute was born in 1984. It has since been responsible for over 20,000 IVF births worldwide, and has made numerous scientific advances in genetics and the reproductive sciences. The Institute has also proven sufficiently successful that in the unlikely event that I, like Bob, wanted to retire to a farm I should be able to do so in reasonable comfort.

Bob and I remained in touch from time to time in the 1980s, and then grew closer in the 90s. He frequently asked me to review new scientific papers to see if they were suitable for publication in the journals he was editing. He crossed the Atlantic on three occasions to give keynote addresses at our Institute including its 10 year anniversary conference in 1994, and did so for the last time in 2004. Bob admired our Institute's scientific achievements, which embrace several hundred peer-reviewed publications. He particularly appreciated our development of a new and powerful method for the prevention of Huntington's disease through a technology known as non-disclosing preimplantation genetic testing, and of course was a strong supporter of applying our method of preconceptual sperm selection (MicroSort) both for the prevention of X-linked genetic diseases and for family gender balancing.

As previously noted, MicroSort was misguidedly obstructed from being made available to patients in the U.K. In the United States, regulatory approval for full patient access to this technology which is unquestionably effective, has already produced approximately 1,300 healthy babies, and can preconceptually reduce gender-related pregnancy terminations has not yet been obtained.

Thus, both in England and the United States, and in many other countries in the world, the introduction of scientifically sound methods for the enhancement of human reproductive alternatives remains inhibited by misunderstanding, bureaucratic fearfulness, and political influences. One hopes this situation will gradually improve. But setbacks continue, as, in a shocking example, IVF technology was banned just a few years ago in Italy.

IVF is a field of medicine that has continued to thrive and advance despite governmental interference and indifference, but with much of the progress being made outside of academic medical centers. On his last visit to America, Bob and I sat together in the beautiful main hall on the second floor of Washington's Cosmos Club. Taking in the elegant surroundings, Bob smiled and said, "I'm glad to see that you got out of academics and succeeded on your own." I was greatly moved by this complement from a man I admire so much and who had shown the way.

The Nobel Prize which Bob just received was delayed at least 25 years after it should have been made. Numerous scientists, obviously including me, repeatedly stated in public forums that Bob's work deserved this level of recognition. But the Prize was deferred until long after Patrick was dead and unable to share the award, and after Bob had fallen victim to dementia. The prize money, after taxes are paid, will likely be consumed in providing nursing care for Bob over his remaining lifetime. Why was the award, so obviously merited, so long not made? The reasons, in my opinion, had nothing to do with science. Rather, they had everything to do with Bob's reputation as a "controversial" scientist, prolonged opposition from the Vatican which expressed publicly its dismay when the Prize was announced, and the socialistic instincts and academic connections of the Karolinska committee. For these Swedish socialists (and they really are, I have met several of them), Bob had committed the unpardonable sin of becoming prosperous. There have been other examples of this same phenomenon, such as the Nobel committee "overlooking" Herbert Boyer after he discovered certain key techniques of gene splicing and went on to co-found Genentech. Bob had also changed, and was no longer the politically correct left-wing academician he had once been when at Cambridge University. Then also he had the temerity to speak out forcefully, and sometimes could offend important people. He started a journal which competed with one he had previously edited for a leading European reproductive medicine society. He became a critic of his own government bureaucracies and those of the United States with regard to their policies on some innovative reproductive issues. Such is the list of his major sins.

For these reasons that shameful committee in Stockholm waited so many years to grant a brilliant benefactor of mankind the formal recognition he so obviously had earned. They waited until he was so ill they needed to inform Bob's wife, Ruth, instead of Bob, that he had won the Nobel Prize in Physiology and Medicine. There is an old saying with regard to the law, sometimes attributed to William Gladstone, that justice deferred is justice denied. A Nobel Prize unjustly deferred is also justice denied. It's sad enough to make at least one grown man cry.

I have learned much from Bob Edwards. He personifies the tremendous tenacity, toughness, and persistence which may be needed to accomplish breakthrough science. His life and the experiences of other pioneers in the field of human reproduction illustrate how ignorance, prejudice, politics, and bureaucracy can delay medical research, impede patient access to medical advances, and harm the innovators who make such advances possible. Bob's courage was as important as his brilliance, and neither of these shall I ever forget.

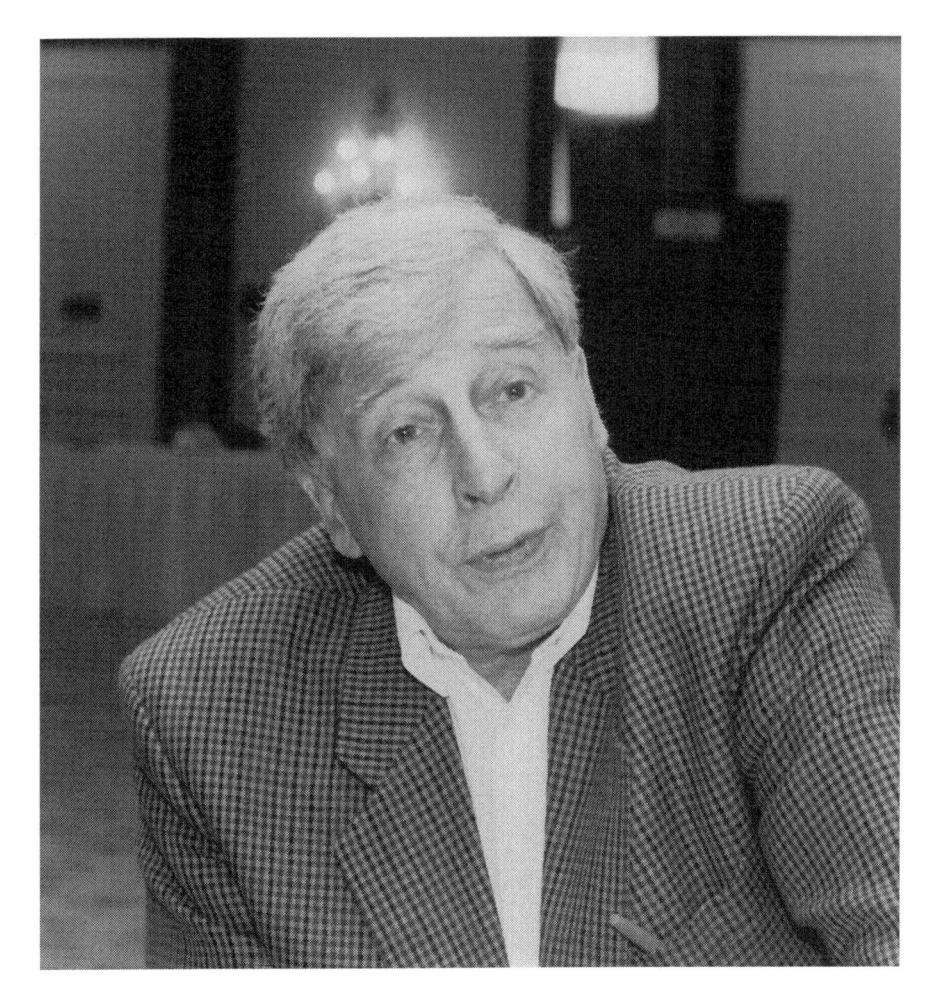

Bob Edwards, Genetics & IVF Institute, 1994

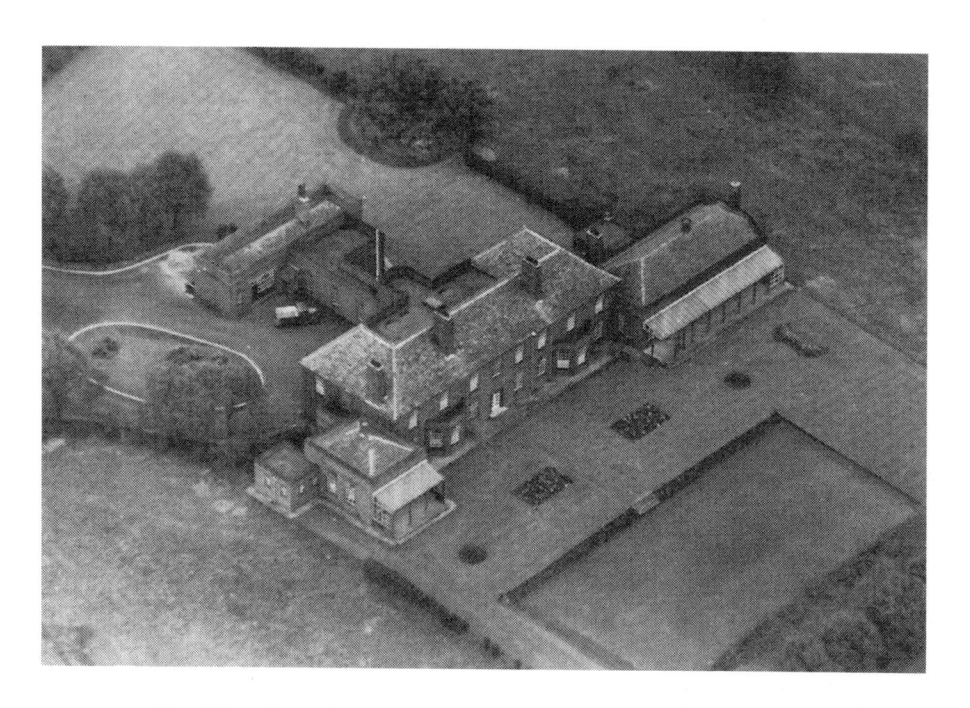

Dr. Kershaw's Cottage Hospital, Royton, c. 1970

Made in the USA
Charleston, SC
01 December 2010